Coconut Oil for Radiant Health & Wellness

An Everyday Use for Healthy Living, Effective Weight Loss, Supple Skin & Glowing Hair – A Quick and Easy Guide

Sabinah Oroge

Dedication

This book is dedicated to:

"All Who Believe in the Efficacy of Coconut Oil for Healthy Living"

Disclaimer and Terms of Use

The information provided in this book is for general information and education purposes only. While the author has tried to keep the information correct and authentic, the contents are not intended to replace, prescribe, diagnose or treat any illness or disease. It is recommended that you consult your doctor if you have any health concerns you may wish to address.

TABLE OF CONTENTS

INTRODUCTION

A few years back, let's take a decade for example; people's point of view on coconut oil was negative. The popular trend then was about the toxic saturated fats in the coconut oil and their harmful effects on the body. So it was avoided at that time, and coconut oil was tagged a "villain". That notion of coconut oil was absurd. Why? The information I am going to share with you, will make all those ideas and concepts on coconut oil baseless and unjust.

Do you know that coconut oil is a major ingredient in baby products because of its soothing properties and vitamins in its composition, which are also present in breast milk? Do you know that early stage cancer patients and Alzheimer's patients are treated with coconut oil because of its medicinal properties? Do you know that Food and Drug Administration (FDA) includes coconut oil in the list of safe foods? Do you know how much potential it has to burn excess fat in the body? Do you know it is enough to treat major health problems? Do you know in the testimonies of the Ayurvedic Medical Journals dated four centuries back, coconut oil and health benefits were found and extremely likable at that time for remedies? Do you know tropical countries and South Asian countries call the coconut palm tree as "The Tree of Life"? Then how come the notion that coconut oil is bad?

Why was coconut oil publicized as unhealthy? The two major reasons I have found after tons of study, is the lack of detailed research on coconut oil and even the little research done was not being shared with others. No one knows much about the miracles of coconut oil and its benefits until recently when people are becoming more aware of the truth about it. What actually stopped people from using coconut oil in their diet were two words, 'Saturated Fats'? Saturated fats meant heart problems and obesity, which ultimately lead to an unhealthy body.

This book is set to share amazing facts about coconut oil, which will shed some more light on the benefits and efficacy of coconut oil. Now, it is very essential to develop correct and proper understanding about saturated fats.

The saturated fats present in the coconut oil are actually medium chain. It is actually the long chain fatty acids, which steer coronary problems and weight issues, not medium chain fats. Only few people know the difference between the two types of fatty acids. That is why people shunned the use of tropical oils, mainly coconut oil and palm oil and instead switched to olive oil and soybean oil. Though these oils are nutritious as well, but the fatty acids present in them are actually trans-fats which are toxic to health. The lack of knowledge of the American Standard Association (ASA) and Center for Science in the Public Interest (CSPI) about fatty acids led to several mistakes and health issues.

Soybean and olive oil replaced tropical oils, and a few years later these oils were declared responsible for the high cholesterol levels in the body that increased the number of heart disease patients. Reduce their intake, and the better it is. Moreover, later when ASA and CSPI finally understood and distinguished between long chain and medium chain fatty acids, they failed to inform the public. These further strengthened the misconceptions about tropical oils.

When research on tropical oils started, the media did not pay much attention to it which made coconut oil more unpopular. However, gradually, the truth came out. The examples of the benefits of the healthy coconut oil on the population of the tropical countries could no longer be ignored. Their diets are based on plenty of coconut in the form of palm roots and coconut oil.

Do you know that people living in tropical countries have the lowest rate of heart diseases in the world and have a healthy body? Now compare this situation with the rest of the world where trans-fats are consumed and very little coconut oil and then their health issues. This does not mean that fats in coconut oil do not affect cholesterol levels. Medium chain fatty acids have a neutral effect on blood cholesterol level than the long chain fatty acids. This example can reflect the beneficial health effects in the morbidity and mortality of the tropical population who consume a large amount of coconut oil.

The other encouraging and positive effects of coconut oil are discussed below. Keep reading and discover this hidden treasure that will surely change your life.

Why You Should Read This Book and Take Action Thereafter?
This book presents in an easy to read manner information on:

i) Why coconut oil is the newest kid on the block and why it is called the super food.
ii) What coconut oil is, the basic facts and constituents.
iii) The mind blowing facts and data to support that coconut oil is healthy and have positive impacts on the health of individuals.
iv) The nutritional information to help in evaluating the intake of calories on the consumption of coconut oil.
v) The benefits of coconut oil to the entire family.
vi) Easy to make coconut oil recipes for either cooking or baking.
vii) Recipes for homemade body care products for everyday use.
viii) How coconut oil makes your body healthy by treating major and common ailments.
ix) The positive impact of coconut oil on the beauty and weight of individuals.

Fatty acids and oils are organic substances, which are composed of carbon, oxygen and hydrogen. When carbon, oxygen and hydrogen are chemically combined with a carboxyl group, a long chain is formed, known as fatty acids. Alternatively, when fats react with water, they break into fatty acids and glycerin. Three chains of fatty acids when they react with glycerol molecule combine to form triglycerides. Molecules of triglycerides are the basis of fats and oil.

The difference in their chemical structure creates alteration in their appearances, properties and functions. There are two types of fatty acids, saturated fatty acids and unsaturated fatty acids.

Saturated fatty acids have no double bond and hence the carbon holds all the hydrogen atoms it can. The common name of saturated fatty acids is natural fatty acids as they are present in meat and dairy products as a result of the process called emulsification. They are recommended to be consumed in a limited amount, as they are responsible for high cholesterol levels in the blood and heart diseases.

Unsaturated fats are of three types. When carbon, hydrogen and oxygen react to the carboxyl group to form fatty acids, bonds are formed in their chemical structure. Omega-3, also known as Linolenic acid and Omega-6, also known as Linoleic acid are essential fatty acids and are necessary to be taken in the diet, as the body cannot create them. Fatty acids with one and more than one double bond are called monounsaturated fatty acids and polyunsaturated fatty acids respectively.

The third type of unsaturated fats are trans-fatty acids. The two sources from which trans-fatty acids come are animal fats and hydrogenated vegetable oil. Since it is mentioned before that animal fatty acids should be consumed less because they raise blood cholesterol level, therefore trans-fatty acids are also to be eaten in small portions.

Oil is composed of hydrogen, carbon and oxygen and they are formed when these three elements react with the carboxyl group. Oil is more saturated with unsaturated fatty acids and that is why oil is liquid at room temperature. As the proportion of saturated fats increases, then oil turns solid. Therefore, the state of oil depends on the two conditions.

There is no denying the fact that coconut oil is rich in harmless saturated fat, fatty acids and lipids. What stopped people before using coconut oil in their diet was the risk of heart diseases that are associated with an increase in blood cholesterol level. First, cholesterol is not the only reason of heart diseases. Secondly, there are two types of cholesterol levels in the blood, LDL (bad) and HDL (good). When there is an increase in LDL cholesterol, this may lead to heart diseases. To prove that coconut oil does not cause heart diseases, medical records were compared of both western and tropical populations. It was found that western people consuming sunflower and olive oil have high risk of heart diseases than tropical people consuming coconut oil diet.

An experiment that was carried out among Filipino women, indicated a linkage between taking coconut oil and higher levels of HDL (good cholesterol) when compared with those who did not have coconut oil as part of their daily diet. Moreover, blood coagulation was also improved among the candidates who ate coconut oil therefore decreasing the risk of death by heart attack.

Studies on coconut oil revealed that the fatty acids in coconut oil have a potential to cure brain disorders such as Epilepsy, Alzheimer and seizures, as well as boosting memory also. When drugs failed to treat Alzheimer's disease, coconut oil was used as a natural remedy for the treatment and the results came out surprisingly successful. At the Alzheimer's Institute of Florida, 65 Alzheimer patients were put on medication of coconut oil, while others were put on commercial drugs. It was shown that some cases, which were not at the severe stage of Alzheimer disease, showed greater improvement than those on drugs, by reversing the symptoms of Alzheimer and making memory better.

Coconut oil is enriched with ketone energy and cholesterol, which are a great alternative of energy to the brain. In the same manner, healthy saturated fat in coconut oil treats and reverses the symptoms of diabetes and so far has effectively been used to cure type 2 diabetes. Coconut oil improves body insulin by curbing hunger and the craving for sweets. Population study carried out in the tropical island of South Pacific disclosed that in those that shunned food high in coconut oil, the rate of cases of diabetes increased. As coconut oil improves brain function which includes the hypothalamus region as well, it also cures type 1diabetes by giving rest to pancreas to self-heal itself to secrete insulin in the blood, meanwhile coconut oil provides necessary glucose and energy to the body as it is an instant source of energy.

Coconut oil also helps with weight loss. It is a natural source of fatty acids, which burns unwanted fat in the abdominal cavity and ultimately gets rid of a very common health problem namely obesity. In a small study to prove the relationship of coconut oil with weight loss, the waistline of obese men and women were found to reduce significantly when coconut oil was used as food. Moreover, it was tested that the more healthy men consume coconut oil at breakfast, the less they consume calories during lunch, and therefore coconut oil reduces their hunger. Another daily use of coconut oil which has become popular is to use it as a moisturizer to treat dry scalp and rough hairs for its improvement and to prevent them from any damage. A clinical trial revealed that the dry skin of selected individuals became hydrated and soft when treated with coconut oil massages.

Recently, coconut oil is being tested as biodiesel, lubricant and transformer oil. This has so far been successful in the Philippines, Samoa and other tropical countries where coconut oil is used to fuel vehicle engines and power generators as well. Further researches are still on to process coconut oil as fuel for electricity generation.

CHAPTER 3 - WHAT IS COCONUT OIL?

Coconut oil is an edible oil used in cooking, baking and frying, and in other applications including medical and pharmaceutical industries. Since coconut oil contains more saturated fat, therefore it is solid at room temperature. However, in tropical countries because of the temperature, it is normally found in liquid form. Coconut oil is extracted from the coconut shells of the palm trees using fire, sunlight or kiln. It is estimated that 1440kg of coconuts will produce about 70 liters of coconut oil.

Coconut oil is stable and non-volatile, thus has a long shelf life. As mentioned earlier in this book, that due to the presence of saturated fats and the misconceptions and lack of knowledge about saturated fats, people were advised to consume less coconut oil in their diet. However, with the increase in research and the sharing of findings, now coconut oil is termed as "miracle oil" and is used as a super food daily. These fatty acids are not at all harmful to the body and neither cause any health problems.

a) Basic Facts

This tropical oil comes with a long list of health benefits some of which are listed below.

i)   Coconut oil is made up of medium chain fatty acids, which are healthy forms of saturated fatty acids. At first, people had concepts that saturated fats are harmful to the body as they increase the risk of heart diseases. But that is not true, it is a long chain saturated fatty acid which is associated with coronary diseases than the medium chain saturated fats and that is why they have a neutral effect on the blood cholesterol levels as well.

ii)   Medium chain fatty acids are easily broken down in the liver and converted into energy in the cells, rather than being stored like other fats. That is why it is used for energy to perform vital activities for metabolism. In other words, coconut oil is a great source of instant energy. A test was carried out, in which participants who consumed coconut oil burned more kilojoules of energy than those who did not consume or consumed less coconut oil.

iii) In 2009, in a study on coconut oil on women, it was found that participants who consumed coconut oil daily, lost weight, specifically, their abdominal fat reduced than those women who did not consume coconut oil.

iv) Coconut oil eases digestion. It has anti-microbial properties that fight microbes present in the gut, tummy bugs, parasites and other germs that cause poor digestion. Moreover, the presence of lauric acid aids anti-bacterial, anti-viral and anti-fungal properties in the coconut oil, boosts immune system by killing toxic microbes, harmful pathogens and viruses.

v) Occurrence of antioxidants in coconut oil gives it a soothing and hydrating property; that is why coconut oil is highly used to treat skin-aging problems. It has been found to heal connective tissues. This makes coconut oil a perfect natural ingredient to use in beauty care products and baby products as a healer to treat acne, baby rashes, bruises, dry scalp, cracked lips, and for hydrating skin and massaging purposes.

vi) Medium chain fatty acids are very small molecules; they are quickly absorbed into the cells and converted into energy. This process improves insulin sensitivity and therefore reduces the risks of *diabetes mellitus* in the body.

vii) Coconut oil is best for cooking at high temperatures. This is because of the medium chain fatty acids, which give the high smoking temperature. Coconut oil is a great alternative for oil and butter and especially for vegans who do not eat any dairy products. Those who want a high protein, vegan and gluten free delicious diet, should opt for coconut oil in their daily cooking.

b) Nutritional Information

1 tablespoon of coconut oil contains 116 calories from 14 grams of fat, among which 11.7g fats are saturated, 0.8g from monounsaturated fats and 0.2g polyunsaturated fats. It also contains 243 milligrams of omega-6 fatty acids.

The remaining proportion consists of antioxidant and phenolic compounds like iron, Vitamins E and K. Antioxidants heal the body cells, repair connective tissues, free the skin from radicals and toxins. Coconut oil does not contain cholesterol, carbohydrates, sugars and protein.

CHAPTER 4 - DIFFERENT KINDS OF COCONUT OIL

Coconut oil is now getting the deserved attention and popularity. This tropical oil comes in four forms.

i)   Pure

The pure form of coconut oil is commonly known as virgin or extra-virgin coconut oil. Pure coconut oil is extracted from the shell of coconuts. The meat present in the shell of the coconut undergoes either the wet milling process or through the drying process. The most common method for the extraction of coconut oil is a quick drying method. This method first dries the meat and is mechanically expressed to extract the oil. While, wet milling extraction method involves expression of coconut milk from the fresh coconut meat.

The coconut oil is then extracted by separating the milk using enzymes or centrifuge. These two extraction processes are quick and do not involve exposure to high levels of temperature. Therefore, the flavors and odors of coconut oil are retained. Pure coconut oil is also known as unrefined oil, it is costly as it is not chemically changed and therefore is more superior to the refined oil.

ii)   Refined

The coconut oil, which is bleached and deodorized, is known as refined oil which is extracted from the copra (dried coconut meat). Some industries use chemical solvent to extract as much oil as possible. The oil obtained is purified to remove contamination during the drying process. The oil is then exposed to high level of temperature to remove the flavors and odors in the coconut oil, thereby making it tasteless and without odors. To prolong the life of the refined oil, coconut oil is mixed with sodium hydroxide. Some industries partially hydrogenate refined oil which leads to the oil containing trans-fats. Therefore, this form of coconut oil should be consumed less as trans-fats are responsible for the rise in blood cholesterol levels. Refined coconut oil is used for cooking at higher temperatures, without adding any flavor of coconut to the dish, soap making and bathing products.

iii) Fermented

Fermented coconut oil is the least consistent and has more variability than other forms of coconut oil. This process of fermented coconut oil starts from grating coconut meat, which is then pressed to extract the coconut cream. The coconut cream is placed in a bucket and allowed to ferment at almost 98.6 degrees F, where protein emulsion is broken down by enzymes and bacteria to separate it into four different layers. The four different layers are protein curd, which is at the top, followed by the coconut oil layer and another layer of protein curd, and the last layer is a vinegar layer. To obtain coconut oil, the layer of protein curd and acids of fermentation are removed by filters as much as possible. The high proportion of moisture in the fermented oil is evaporated by heating to 212 degrees F for several hours. Fermented oil is not commercially used because it has a short life span. The remaining acids of fermentation make the oil to taste awful and it also gives a burning sensation in the throat after swallowing.

iv) Organic

Organic coconut oil is extracted from the palm trees that grow on organic feed in the soil, without any addition of fertilizer and spraying of pesticides in the soil. It is the purest and best form of coconut oil. Organic coconut oil is rare to find in the market and very expensive. However, the organic coconut oil, if available, is mainly organic virgin coconut oil.

i) How to Make Coconut Oil at Home

Following are two simple methods to make fresh virgin coconut oil at home, without the use of any machinery or chemical. You just need mature coconuts to begin the process.

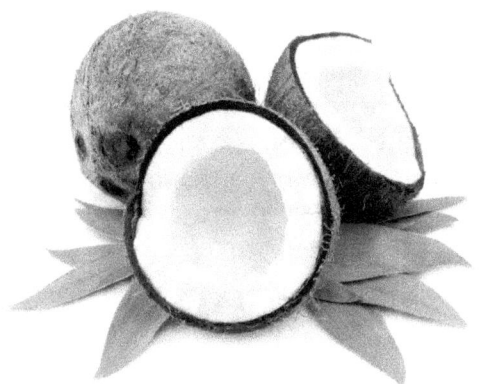

a) Heating process:

The method begins with obtaining the coconut milk. Remove the outer shells of three coconuts and drain the coconut water in a separate container. Grate the meat of the coconut and place the grated meat in the mesh bag. Now hold the bag very tightly and use palms to press and squeeze it. A semi-thick liquid will come out of it, which is called coconut milk. Dip the bag in the coconut water container and press it tightly again to extract more coconut milk. Add water to further extract the milk from the pulp.

Place the coconut milk in a deep pan and heat over low flame, stirring frequently. As the coconut milk reaches to a thick consistency, the oil will start to separate from the milk and the moisture will evaporate. Continue cooking until the water completely evaporates and coconut oil and mush are left behind. Switch off the flame and take the pan off the stove. Leave it aside to cool, pour the oil into a cute glass jar and store.

b) Fermentation:
Obtain coconut milk as mentioned in the above method. Now mix the coconut water with coconut milk, pour into a glass jar and keep aside for a day at room temperature. After one day, you will see coconut oil floating on the water. Filter the oil, it should be colorless or pale yellow in color. Store the oil in a glass or plastic jar.

ii)   **How to Store Coconut Oil**
Coconut oil changes its state as the temperature fluctuates. Store coconut oil is either in liquid or semi-solid form in a glass or plastic container. Just make sure to keep the jar away from direct exposure to sunlight. Coconut oil can be stored in the fridge for maximum of two years. When in the fridge, it will be in solid form. Just heat it in the oven for a few seconds before using it. But at room temperature, about 25 degree Celsius, coconut oil stays liquid.

CHAPTER 6 - WHAT TO LOOK FOR WHEN BUYING COCONUT OIL?

With the understanding of the benefits of the fatty acids present in coconut oil, the market is now filled with various kinds and brands of coconut oil. The question now is, which one of them is best to buy?

The purpose for which you want to use the coconut oil for will determine which one to buy. For example, virgin coconut oil is great for beauty care because of its moisturizing properties, whereas refined coconut oil is great for cooking purposes at high temperatures.

Following are some tips to help you to pick the best coconut oil.

a) Purpose of Buying Coconut Oil - If you are planning to consume coconut oil directly without adding it in the diet, then choose virgin coconut oil. Virgin coconut oil is not processed and hence contains the natural odor and taste of coconut. It is made from fresh coconuts, but the processing method may vary. Virgin coconut oil is used less in cooking and more for a healthy body. Virgin oil brands vary in flavors of coconut oil, from intense to mild. Therefore, choose virgin coconut oil that has mild coconut taste, as the intense coconut taste in the oil is obtained from being exposed to heat for a long time.

b) If you are planning to cook with coconut oil, then purchase refined type. Nevertheless, refined coconut oil has many brands as well. Avoid coconut oil that is hydrogenated and partially hydrogenated, as they contain trans-fat, which may lead to heart and cholesterol problems. Choose refined oil that is refined using chemical free methods.

c) Extraction Method - The extraction method actually improves the coconut oil taste. In a few extraction methods, coconut oil is heated to a high temperature, (which is not good) though coconut oil is stable at higher temperatures. However, the higher the temperature, the more intense the flavor of the oil, which should be avoided. Therefore, choose coconut oil, which is extracted through centrifuge method or through the expeller pressed method. In these methods, the oil is exposed to less heat, therefore would have a mild flavor.

d) Budget – Coconut oil, especially virgin coconut oil is pricey. In order to buy this healthy coconut oil and save money as well, always buy coconut oil in bulk. The stability and long shelf life of coconut oil at room temperature or either storing in fridge eliminate any doubts and dangers that are raised in buying coconut oil in bulk. Though before buying a great deal of coconut oil, it is advisable to first try a small amount and check if it is suitable for your purpose as in taste and odor.

Coconut oil has been found to be a natural shield to protect from bacteria, fungi, and viruses. Coconut oil has hundreds of daily uses. From treating babies for rashes and soft baby skin, to healing damaged tissues e.g. scalps and cracked lips, to dry hairs, for body scrub to nourish the skin, for a fresh deodorant and soap, for cooking and many more.

It is not possible to list all the uses of coconut oil under the present title of this book. However, find below uses to which coconut oil can be put to.

Here are the wonderful ways to incorporate this resourceful oil in your diet, beauty care and for a radiant and healthy body.

a) By the Entire Family
i)   Babies

Coconut oil is a natural healer and nourishing oil for babies. The small molecules of the coconut oil is easily absorbed through the skin into the tissues and cells and therefore heals damaged skin such as baby acne and diaper rashes. Put coconut oil lightly on the affected areas and see the magic. Not only this, apply coconut oil on the bruises and treat them along with swelling and redness. Coconut oil also stops itching from the bites of bugs and soothes the burning sensations caused by bug bites, chicken pox illness etc. Use coconut oil as a baby massage oil and lotion for the body and moisturizer for the dry skin.

ii)   Older Children

The biggest problem in older children is lice problem. Mix apple cider vinegar and coconut oil together and apply it liberally on the scalp to kill head lice. Apply coconut oil on injuries to heal the damaged tissues. Coconut oil is a natural conditioner for hairs. Add in children's diets to boost their brain activity. Take a teaspoon of coconut oil to treat sore throat and add in tea to treat cold or flu. It is also immensely useful in the treatment of acne in teenagers.

iii)   Mum for Her Skin, Hair, Make Up Remover, Facial Scrub

The antioxidant property in coconut oil helps in fighting germs and treating bacterial, fungal and viral infections on the skin. It does wonders to the sensitive woman's skin and hair. A very common use of coconut oil is as a moisturizer; it hydrates and softens dry skin. All beauty products contain virgin coconut oil as the main ingredients for beauty care. Coconut oil is easily absorbed in the cell and repairs them along while providing essential nourishment to the skin by cleansing it. Massage body with a tablespoon of coconut oil after bath and relax yourself. Coconut oil is great as a natural conditioner and makes hair shine and strengthens their growth, resulting in thick, wavy hairs. In the next Chapter, you will find some easy homemade beauty care coconut oil products.

iv) Dad for Shaving

The greatest benefit a man can get from coconut oil is during shaving. Coconut oil will make the skin soft and moisturized, all ready for the razor to glide smoothly without any danger of burning sensations or cuts. You will find in the next Chapter, the recipe for homemade chemical free shaving cream.

b) Treatment of Acne

Acne is an infamous and most common problem among people of all ages. It is very embarrassing especially for teenagers. It leaves marks on the face and not everyone is lucky to get rid of these marks. Coconut oil is a natural remedy for the painful and irritable acne.

Acne is actually an infection of the sebum glands on the skin that secrete oil to moisturize the skin to prevent the skin from drying. Sebum gland is clogged by bacteria when the secretion of oil increases. This causes oily look on the skin and the appearance of pimples. Removing pimples leaves the pores open that are blocked by dirt and hence bacteria in the environment cause infection in these pores. This results in the combination of burning sensation, swelling, redness and irritable pain and itching, or in another word 'Acne'.

In this situation, coconut oil comes to save the skin. The anti-bacterial property and anti-microbial agents in the coconut oil fight the bacteria and covers the pores with an acid layer to stop infection. Anti-inflammatory property in the coconut oil creates a soothing effect on the skin and relieves the pain by healing the wounds.

When the acne areas are treated with coconut oil directly, the fatty acids present in it cover the open pores of acne to protect the area from viral and other infections and curb inflammation.

c) Caring for the Teeth: Oil Pulling Routine

Oil pulling is actually an old dental hygiene technique involved with the cleansing of the mouth by drawing out toxin from the body by swishing oil in the mouth for about 15-20 minutes in the morning. This method effectively improves oral health and if the mouth is clean, then the whole body is clean. It has been found that coconut oil effectively kills the bacteria called *Streptococcus Mutans*, which are responsible for causing cavities in the teeth. This method is the same as the cleansing of the skin.

Oil pulling, amongst other things has been found to whiten the teeth, it prevents bad breath, relieves headache, and strengthens the teeth, gum and jaw. It also acts to generally detoxify the body and it has been established to reduce insomnia.

Following are simple steps for the oil pulling method using coconut oil.

Put two tablespoons of coconut oil into the mouth first thing in the morning. Swish the oil in the mouth for between 15 and 20 minutes.

You will feel saliva mixing with the oil. Spit out the coconut oil into the trash can, **NOT** into the sink (it could block the sink when the oil solidifies).

Clean your teeth as you normally do. Or in the alternative, Use homemade coconut toothpaste to brush your teeth.

d) Caring for the Hair

Just like the skin of your face and body, the scalp is also skin, which needs all the care, nourishment and moisturizer to keep the hairs shiny and strong. Take a minute and see the contents in your scalp product, you will definitely find coconut oil.

Coconut oil has a soothing effect on the scalp when massaged with it. Add a few drops of your favorite essential oil in it and moisturize your dry, itchy skin of the scalp. The anti-bacterial property in coconut oil will fight the bacterial and fungal infections of the scalp, and will reduce dandruff and hair loss, and repair scalp tissues.

Take a 5-7 tablespoon of coconut oil in a bowl, the quantity depends on the thickness and length of the hair. Warm it for 30 seconds in microwave and massage your scalp and roots of the hair with it.

The proper way to give the scalp a massage is by applying coconut oil in one-inch portion of hairs so that every hair and portion of the scalp is treated evenly. After applying coconut oil, rub the fingertips on the scalp in circular motion for 10 minutes and let coconut oil remain in the hair for 1 hour before washing.

And in your next hair wash, you will feel your hair glossy, soft and silky. Infants should as well be given a massage of coconut oil on the scalp to stimulate hair growth.

e) Prevents Stretch Marks

Stretch marks are caused by the stretching of the skin. This may occur during pregnancy, puberty, during weight gain etc. By keeping the skin moisturized with coconut oil, can help prevent stretch marks. Coconut oil because of its nourishing property provides moisture and elasticity which goes right into the skin. Massaging some onto the area daily will be of tremendous help. When applied 2-3 times daily during pregnancy keeps stretch marks at bay.

f) Vapor Rub for Stuffy Nose and Chest

Coconut oil mixed with a few drops of peppermint essential oil or eucalyptus oil can be applied beneath the nose and chest to clear the stuffiness and you get a relief.

g) Nipple Cream for Breast Feeding Mothers

The soreness and pain of cracked nipples especially for nursing mothers can be reduced to the barest minimum by applying coconut oil on the affected nipples after breast feeding.

h) Keeps Leaves of Plants Shinning
To keep the leaves of your indoor plants looking healthy and dust-free, rub some coconut oil on them. Repeat this as often as needed

i) Lights a Campfire
A safe way to start a campfire is by assembling cotton balls soaked in coconut oil and lighting them.

j) Inhibits Cold Sores Virus
The herpes simplex virus causes cold sore which can be quite painful. Coconut oil may not be able to wipe out the virus, but it can prevent the spread. The lauric acid in coconut oil prevents the virus from reproducing and multiplying. Just apply coconut oil on the sore many times a day.

k) Cleans Furniture
Condition and clean wooden kitchen utensils and furniture with coconut oil by applying it generously for a glossy look.

l) Treats Athlete's Foot
Apply coconut oil daily to treat athlete's foot. The anti-fungal property of coconut oil helps in fighting athlete's foot. Before applying it, clean the feet and pat them dry.

m) Removes Rust from Steel Items
In order to get rid of rust on knives, scissors and other household appliances, rub some coconut oil on the affected areas. Leave it for about 2 hours and wipe clean with a soft cloth.

n) Removes Chewing Gum from Surfaces
Often times, the carpet, the furniture and even the hair have chewing gum stuck to them and one is faced with the dilemma of removing or cleaning these items without too much damage. The way out of this is to rub some quantity of coconut oil on the affected part, allow 5-10 minutes and wipe with a piece of cloth. Remove any excess oil with a mild soap and rinse.

o) Relieves Arthritis Pain
Massage some coconut oil into each joint thoroughly 1-2 times a day to relieve the pain caused by arthritis. This helps to ease the discomfort.

p) Soothes Sore Throat

Take ½-1 teaspoon of coconut oil 2- 3 times daily to ease the pain associated with sore throat. It provides a wonderful soothing feeling.

q) Removes Ink Smear

When you are faced with ink smears and smudges on your hand, just rub a little coconut oil over it and wait for about 2 minutes. Wipe off with a dry, clean, cloth.

r) Serves as a Lubricant

Coconut oil is used as a lubricant to remove the squeakiness in door hinges and keep motors in good working position.

s) Heals Cracked Heels

Coconut oil can help soften, smoothen and heal cracked heels. First, remove dead cells by soaking the feet in water and removing the cells by scrubbing with a pumice stone. Rinse and dry the feet. Massage coconut oil using the finger tips. Repeat twice daily until the heels are completely healed and smooth.

t) Relieves Constipation

If you are constipated, take a tablespoon of coconut oil in the morning on an empty stomach to keep your digestive system running in a more efficient way.

u) Releases a Jammed Zipper

When you find it difficult to zip up your skirts, pants or any of your clothing, apply a bit of coconut oil on the jammed zipper, rub it in, and it should slide with ease.

Adding coconut oil in the diet is not only beneficial for health, it is also used for a variety of other things like the natural beauty of skin and hairs.

Recently, coconut oil has become extremely popular and a preferable ingredient for making skin care products. The main reasons behind this popularity are the properties inherent in coconut oil.

Coconut oil contains antioxidant, antibacterial and anti-fungal properties which provide nourishment to the skin and hold remedy for any skin problem, be it for anti-aging, wrinkles, acne, dry lips and scalp, even for baby rashes. Following are some beauty products having coconut oil as the main ingredient for skin and hair care.

i) Ointment for Diaper Rash, Baby Wash and Baby Lotion

Coconut oil is nourishing oil for infants. It is absorbed in the body very easily and due to its healing property, it restores damaged tissues and that is why coconut oil is highly recommended now to treat rashes on the infant's body. It is also used to treat dry skin on the infant's scalp and to strengthen the hair. The most common and traditional use of coconut oil is the massage of the baby's body. To make a soothing baby massage cream

Ingredients:

½ cup coconut oil

¼ cup olive oil

7 drops of lavender essential oil (or any other oil)

Method:

In a bowl, place coconut oil and olive oil together and using electric mixer, whip until it has a light and airy consistency for 6-8 minutes. Add in essential oil and whip for 2 more minutes. Spoon the cream in a cute plastic container

Coconut oil is used for healing. For treating baby acne, dab the affected areas with coconut oil twice a day until it vanishes completely. Rub coconut oil onto the gums, as a natural remedy to effectively reduce the pain during teething of babies and for the growth of teeth.

Coconut oil is used as a main ingredient in the baby diaper cream. This cream successfully prevents baby's nappy rash. Follow the recipe below for the homemade baby diaper cream. Use this cream with diapers.

Ingredients:

½ cup coconut oil

¼ cup shea butter

1 tablespoon beeswax pastilles

2 tablespoons Fermented Cod Liver Oil

2 tablespoons zinc oxide powder

1 tablespoon bentonite clay

Method:
Place a saucepan over low flame; add shea butter, coconut oil and beeswax together. Measure an inch of water and pour in the pan. Let the contents in the pan melt. Switch off the flame and then add remaining ingredients. Stir and allow the mix to cool. Continue stirring until the mixture completely cools down. Put it in a container, cover it tightly and store in a dry place at room temperature for use.

ii)   Chemical free Shaving Cream

Ingredients:

2/3 cup coconut oil

2/3 cup shea butter

¼ cup olive oil

15 drops of lavender essential oils or your favorite essential oil

2 tablespoons of baking soda

Method:

Place pan over medium heat and place coconut oil and shea butter in it. Stir and allow to melt. Switch off the flame and pour in olive oil. Transfer the mixture into a mixing bowl, and add essential oil. Stir and keep it in the fridge to harden, for one to two hours. Then remove from the fridge and let it rest to soften lightly. Now add baking soda and use an electric mixer to beat until airy and fluffy. Store it in a glass container and keep it in a cool, dark place.

iii) Hand /Body Cream

Coconut oil cream is best especially in the dry season. The coconut oil hand cream keeps hands from drying and moisturizes hands and even feet for the whole day. This best moisturizer hand cream works effectively. This cream remains soft throughout the cold months. If it's in a liquid state, it can be placed in the fridge to solidify.

Ingredients

1/4 cup coconut oil

1/8 cup shea butter

1/8 cup cocoa butter

1 tablespoon sweet almond oil

7 drops lavender oil

Method:

Place a bowl in a pot of hot water over low heat and add coconut oil, shea and cocoa butter together. Heat until all the contents in the bowl is melted. Mix well and switch off the flame and mix all together. Add the sweet almond and lavender oil, stir well to combine everything. Use an electric hand mixer to whip the mixture until it is fluffy. Store in a plastic jar at room temperature. Apart from using it as a hand cream, it can also be used on the whole body.

iv) **Moisturizing Hand Cream:**

Ingredients:

¼ cup coconut oil

½ cup olive oil

¼ cup beeswax

2 tablespoons shea butter

7 drops Vanilla Extract

Method:

Place a saucepan over low heat and add coconut oil, olive oil, beeswax, shea butter and vanilla extract. Heat until contents in the pan melts. Mix well and switch off the flame. Transfer the oil mix in a jar and store at room temperature.

v) **Lemon Whipped Hand Scrub:**

Ingredients:

½ cup coconut oil

1 tablespoon olive oil

2 tablespoons aloe vera gel

15 drops lime essential oil

15 drops lemon essential oil

Method:

In a medium size mixing bowl, add coconut oil, olive oil, aloe vera, lime essential and lemon essential oil together. Use electric mixture to whip the contents for 8-10 minutes until light and airy consistency is obtained. Spoon the whipped the mix into a cute glass or plastic jar. Store in the refrigerator.

vi)　**Body Lotion**

Coconut oil, even in solid state, is a perfect light lubricant that can spread liberally all over the body. Store it in a bottle in the washroom cabinet and rub it lightly right after the shower, the warmth of the body will melt the oil and it will sink well into the body. The result will be fresh, baby soft skin. Moreover, coconut oil massaged all over the body will leave tropical fragrance that will help you remain fresh all day long.

Ingredients:

1 cup coconut oil

A few drops of essential oil of your choice

Method:

Do not melt the coconut oil. Place coconut and essential oil in the mixing bowl and whipped for 7-8 minutes using electric mixer until light and fluffy. Place the mixture in an attractive glass or plastic container and cover tightly. Store at room temperature.

vii) **Whipped Orange & Peppermint Body Butter:**

Ingredients:

¼ cup coconut oil

6 tablespoons shea butter

2 tablespoons cocoa butter

¼ cup almond oil

10 drops orange essential oil

8 drops peppermint oil

Method:

Heat saucepan over low heat. Place shea butter, cocoa butter and coconut oil together. Heat until contents in the pan melt. Mix well, switch off the flame and let it cool for about 30 minutes. Transfer to a bowl and add essential oils. Mix well and let it cool sufficiently for 20-25 minutes in the fridge. Check the oil mix and as soon the outer edge of the oil mix solidifies, use electric mixer to whip until a light and airy consistency is obtained. Place this whipped mixture in an attractive glass container.

viii) **Vanilla & Sugar Body Scrub:**

Ingredients:

½ cup solid coconut oil,

1 cup white sugar

Seeds from 2 vanilla bean pods

Method:

Place solid coconut oil in a bowl. Use electric mixer to whip into a light and airy consistency for 8-10 minutes. The blender can also be used as an alternative, do not forget to scrap the sides. Now add sugar and vanilla seeds and continue whipping for a couple of minutes. Transfer this mixture into a cute glass or plastic container.

ix) Night Cream

Coconut oil night cream is an effective cleansing. For best results apply it a few minutes before the bed time. Smear on face and neck, soon you will notice a fresh soft skin.

Ingredients:

1 tablespoon coconut oil

3 tablespoons shea butter

3 drops tea tree oil

Method:

In a mixing bowl, place coconut oil and shea butter, mix everything together. Stir in tea tree oil and mix well. Use the back of the spoon to mix the coconut oil, shea butter and tea tree oil. Put the mixture in a plastic container and use as often as you desire.

x) Nourishing Night Scrub:

Ingredients:

1 tablespoon coconut oil

2 tablespoons raw honey

¼ cup sea salt

¼ cup organic sugar

1 tablespoon lemon juice

Method:

In a medium size mixing bowl, add coconut oil and honey together and mix using back of the spoon. In another bowl, add the remaining ingredients and mix very well until crumbly. Pour this mix over coconut-honey mixture and stir until well combined. Spoon the cream in a cute plastic or glass container and store at room temperature.

xi) **Lip Balm**

Coconut oil is a natural hydrating agent for chapped lips. Scoop some coconut oil in a spare tiny plastic box and smudge it with fingers on the lips throughout the day. Make this homemade lip balm and gift some to your friends or family members.

Ingredients

1 tablespoon coconut oil

1 tablespoon beeswax, grated

1 teaspoon olive oil

Method:

Place a saucepan over low heat, add coconut oil, beeswax and olive oil. Heat until contents in the pan melt. Mix well and switch off the flame. Pour the mixture in the storage container or tin and let it cool completely before using on the lips.

Tips:

The oil selection depends on the color of the lip, olive oil gives faint yellow color into lip balm and red palm oil leave orange color to lips, a dash of beet root powder gives red color to lips whereas to leave brown color on lips, add one quarter teaspoon of cocoa powder.

xii)   **Natural Lip Balm:**

2 tablespoons coconut oil

1 tablespoon beeswax, grated

1 tablespoon shea butter

7 drops lemon oil

Method:

Place a saucepan over low heat and add coconut oil, beeswax and shea butter. Heat until contents in the pan melt. Mix well and switch off the flame. Add in lemon oil and stir well. Pour the mixture using dropper in the storage container or tin and let it cool completely before using on the lips.

xiii) **Healing Lip Balm:**

1 tablespoon virgin coconut oil

1 tablespoon grated beeswax or beeswax pastilles

A dash of organic raw honey

2 vitamin-E capsules

Method:

Place a saucepan over low heat and add coconut oil, beeswax and honey. Heat until contents in the sauce have melted. Mix well and switch off the flame. Open the vitamin E capsules, pour the contents into mixture and stir well. Pour the whole mixture in the storage container or tin and let it cool completely before using on the lips. This lip balm is amazing for healing cracked lips.

xiv) Deodorant for Sensitive Skin

The use of coconut oil deodorant is becoming very popular among guys and girls. Just follow the recipe below, and make your own scented deodorant. Use fingers to rub under armpits before dressing.

Ingredients:

1/3 cup coconut oil

2 tablespoons baking soda

10 drops of sweet orange oil

5 drops of cinnamon oil

1/3 cup arrowroot powder

Method:

In a medium size-mixing bowl, add coconut oil, baking soda and arrowroot together. Mix and cream the contents using the back of the spoon, until it reaches to deodorant like consistency. Add sweet orange and cinnamon oil and mix. Now transfer this mixture in a cute small container. Store at room temperature.

xv) Coconut Oil Soap

Ingredients:

33 ounces of coconut oil

4.96 ounces of lye

12.5 ounces of water

1 ounce rose essential oil or any essential oil of your choice

Method:

Before following up the method to make the soap, check the temperature of the coconut oil which should be 76 degrees C.

Place a saucepan on a low flame and add coconut oil. Heat oil until it has completely melted. Switch off the flame.

Measure the coconut oil which should be 33 ounces and pour into a crock pot.

Add measured water in a separate bowl and in another separate bowl, pour in the lye.

Now gradually but slowly add lye into the bowl of water (**DO NOT ADD WATER TO THE LYE**). Be careful with this process because of the lye; do not allow it to touch your skin.

Use a metal spoon to stir. This will produce a cloudy white mixture that that is very hot.

It is better to cover your mouth to prevent inhaling fumes during this mixing process. Wait until the mixture cools down and is clear.

Use rubber or plastic gloves to handle the bowl, as it will be very warm.

Now carefully add the lye-water mixture into the crock pot. Then mix until it looks like a pudding consistency.

Switch on the flame to medium and place the crock pot. Cover the pot and cook the soap mixture until it bubbles.

Let it rise and cook for about 50 minutes until it has Vaseline type of consistency.

Switch off the flame and let it stand for a few minutes before checking the soap mixture then add rose essential oil.

Pour the soap mixture in the soap mold and allow to cool until hard and set up for 24-36 hours. Remove from the mold. Your soap is ready for use.

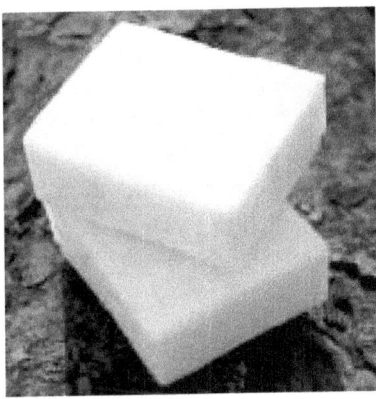

Coconut Oil Soap

i)   Heart Disease

Coconut oil is the latest powerful weapon to fight heart disease. Though saturated fats are responsible for the heart disease and increase their risk, but the saturated fats present in coconut oil made up of medium chain fatty acids and lauric acid, have a negative effect on cholesterol. The variation in cholesterol level leads to heart disease, the more the cholesterol in blood, the greater the chances of heart disease. Studies show that Filipino women who consumed less coconut oil have high cholesterol level in the blood than those who consumed more coconut oil in their diet. Moreover, people in the tropical countries who consumed coconut or coconut oil daily as part of their diet have fewer cases of heart diseases than western countries where unsaturated fats are consumed. Therefore, it is not wrong to say that coconut oil is beneficial, not harmful because of its different effects on blood lipids and cholesterol level.

Another successful research proved that coconut oil lessens heart diseases. Actually, when arteries harden due to formation of plaque, medically known as atherosclerosis, it leads to the narrowing of the blood vessels when plaque starts damaging arteries

Researches are ongoing on coconut oil in relation to heart disease. It is expected that more facts on the efficacy of coconut oil will be revealed.

ii)   Cancer

Virgin coconut oil (unrefined) has been found to contribute to the cure of cancer. The use of coconut oil in medication has led to the decline of cancer patients. Though the decline is low, coconut oil has been found to be effective. Medium chain triglycerides, the major constituent of the fatty acids in coconut oil halt the cancer cell growth by providing fat environment for these cells instead of glucose environment, (which is a source of energy for cancerous cell). Fatty acids when broken down and dissolved in the blood stream, create anti-carcinogenic effects that fight cancerous cells and strengthen the immune system of the body.

iii) Diabetes

Diabetes is an autoimmune ailment in the body, caused either when the body fails to make insulin or when the body fails to respond to the insulin in the blood. Though diabetes can be controlled by taking insulin injection, following strict diet and through exercises, but still there is no cure for this disease. It can be controlled not cured. Now, this widespread disease is treated with coconut oil. How? As we know, coconut oil curbs hunger and the craving of sweetness and maintains a healthy body by improving blood glucose levels. A research in Diabetes Journal tells about an experiment on animals. The test animals that were fed a coconut oil rich diet were found to be healthier than the control group which was not fed with coconut oil. It was found that medium chain fatty acids not only regulated blood sugar level, it also lessened the effect of diabetes on the health of the body. Coconut oil is an instant source of energy and that energy is not in need of insulin to be absorbed by cells. This allows pancreases to heal, as coconut oil has been found to be a natural healer.

iv) Immune System Strengthening

Strengthen your immune system with coconut oil. Antiviral properties and abundance of lauric acid and caprylic acid in coconut oil make it great to boost immunity. Lauric acid cleanses the body by fighting harmful viral infections and pathogen to prevent harmful diseases like cancer, influenza etc. Simply use a tablespoon of coconut oil daily in your diet. Stir in coffee, soups or smoothie and cleanse your body.

v) Allergies

Cure allergies with a tablespoon of coconut oil. Allergies are incurable and are actually symptoms of the body triggered by the immune system to defend the body from infections until removed or calmed. Coconut oil not only protects internally by fighting and killing bacteria through its anti-bacterial, anti-fungal and anti-viral properties, it protects the body externally from the germs and microbes in the environment as well. Coconut oil is a natural allergy relief not only for humans, but also for animals. By simply replacing butter and cooking oil with coconut oil, one can get rid of these irritable allergies.

vi) Cholesterol

Saturated fats cause cholesterol levels to rise up. However, not all types of saturated oils are responsible for the increase in cholesterol level. Saturated fats are made up of fatty acids. The long chain fatty acids are indigestible in the body and hence increase cholesterol level in the body especially bad cholesterol, LDL. Whereas coconut oil is very stable to digest in the body. Hence, it has a neutral effect on the blood cholesterol level and increases good cholesterol in the blood, known as HDL.

vii) Osteoporosis

The medical orthopedic term Osteoporosis means the weakness of bones, which increases the risk of broken bones, even from minor stress. Osteoporosis is very common amongst the old and also men and women of all ages.

Coconut oil nourishes and maintains the health of the bones. A study was carried out on the three groups of mice with a broken bone in each group. Calcium and virgin coconut oil were given to two respective mice groups and the remaining group was the control group. Mice were chosen as test subjects as they show similar response and effects like humans for the bones due to stress, drugs and hormones. The group of mice given coconut oil showed increased level of antioxidants, it reversed the causes of osteoporosis and the result of coconut oil on broken bones was more effective than calcium.

viii) Brain Enhancement (Improvement) in Alzheimer's Disease

Medium chain triglyceride fats in coconut boost the performance of the brain and the treating of serious brain disorders like Alzheimer. This is a groundbreaking discovery about coconut oil, which was tested and showed positive results. The Journal of Neurobiology states that the fatty acids in coconut oil improve mental function along with memory disorders. A group of four Alzheimer patients were tested and were given a dosage of coconut oil, it led to the rise of cholesterol level in the blood and ketone energy which is a great source of energy for the brain. However, glucose is the primary source of energy and nourishment for the brain, but it is only possible when the patient is suffering from diabetes. In this case, ketone energy provides essential energy, resulting in improved mental function and cholesterol recharge to the brain.

The beneficial properties in coconut oil such as anti-oxidants, anti-bacterial, anti-fungal, lauric acid and other make it an exceptional natural medicine to fight health related problems in the body, including hair, heart, kidney, diabetes, digestion, metabolism, hair, skin, stress, obesity and even cancer.

Long chain fatty acids are more difficult to absorb in the body than medium fatty acid chain which are present in the coconut oil. These fats are very easy to digest, break down into finer and simpler molecules called lauric acid that is absorbed in the gut rapidly. Lauric acid is very beneficial and plays a vital role in a healthy body. This promising acid is responsible for boosting metabolism and immunity to fight bacterial and viral diseases. Following are other important valuable health benefits of coconut oil.

i)   Beauty

Coconut oil benefits for beauty are unlimited. The most common advantage is hydrating the skin by using it as a moisturizer. Its small, medium chain fatty acid molecules are easily absorbed through the skin into the cells. They also heal and repair tissues, be it on the face, hands or feet. In this way, coconut oil is great to treat cuticles, cracked lips, bruises or bug bites. Use coconut oil in face pack and masks and see your face in a new glow. The anti-bacterial and anti-fungal properties in the coconut oil effectively treat acne and anti-aging properties smooth the skin. Improve scalp health by giving a soothing massage of coconut oil on dry scalp and root hairs. You will find your scalp moisturizes and dandruff free with strong and soft tresses.

Many pharmaceutical companies now use coconut oil as an ingredient in the production of beauty products.

ii)   Weight Loss

Coconut oil is now widely used in decreasing the weight of the body. This is done by the medium chain fatty acids, which take off excessive weight by burning stored excess fats in the body, mainly in the liver, converting into energy for the vital cell activities and also eases digestion of food.

Since coconut oil improves the metabolic rate, therefore more energy is burned that leads to loss of fat in obese people. It was found in a study that people who include coconut oil in their diet did not increase their weight and their abdominal fat reduced. Replace butter or oil with coconut oil in your recipes.

Quick Ways to Implement Coconut Oil in Your Daily Diet

The direct and simplest ways to implement coconut oil daily is through the diet.

i) The most common way to consume coconut oil in the diet is cooking food with it. Coconut oil is a healthy alternative. Use it to toast bread, as a spread, frying, and bake sweets.

ii) Aside from cooking, coconut oil is used in making healthy smoothies and add freshness in hot beverages like tea, coffee and hot chocolate. Just a tablespoon or two to your beverage, tea or coffee and even to your smoothie and you are on your way to shedding some weight.

iii) Add in healthy soups to enhance flavor.

iv) Coconut oil is an instant source of energy. To prove it, make homemade energy bars using coconut oil instead of with butter.

v) Take a tablespoon of coconut oil first thing in the morning on an empty stomach helps in reducing belly fat.

Incorporating coconut oil in your diet daily and consistently will go a long way in assisting with weight loss especially the reduction of abdominal fat. The next chapter contains cooking and baking recipes where coconut oil is used as the primary cooking or baking oil. These recipes can start you off on a journey towards a radiant health.

CHAPTER 11 – COCONUT OIL RECIPES IN COOKING & BAKING

a) Cooking

Coconut oil is great for cooking healthy and nutritious food. Find below delicious recipes with coconut oil.

i)   SOY AND HONEY CHICKEN:

Serving (s): 4

Ingredients:

4 teaspoons clear honey

4 teaspoons soy sauce

1 lb. boneless, skinless chicken thighs

150g brown rice

pinch of salt

½ teaspoon coconut oil

1 teaspoon black sesame seeds

handful fresh coriander leaves

1 teaspoon pumpkin seeds, chopped

1 tablespoon sesame oil

2 heads of bok choi, halved

Method:

In a medium size mixing bowl, add honey and soy sauce together and stir. Add chicken and mix until coated completely.

Place a deep saucepan over medium flame and place coated chicken in it. Cook for 25 minutes until cooked through and honey-soy glaze is formed.

Meanwhile, heat another pan filled with 5 cups of water. Stir salt and bring water to boil. As the water starts boiling, add rice and bring to boil. Then reduce flame to lower medium and cover the pan. Cook rice for 30 minutes until tender and fluffy. Add coconut oil, sesame seeds and coriander, and stir.

In the meantime, heat sesame oil in a frying pan over medium heat until hot.

Add bak choi in the pan and cook for 5 minutes until leaves are wilted.

Serve bok choi rice on a platter and top with honey chicken.

Nutritional Info:

Carbohydrates: 12.8g

Fats: 6.1g

Protein: 23g

Sugar: 13.4g

ii)   Sautéed Shrimp with Coconut Oil:

Serving (s): 4

Ingredients:

2 ½ tablespoons coconut oil

6 green onions

1 tablespoon fresh ginger

2 garlic cloves

½ teaspoon ground coriander

1 lb. large shrimp, shelled

½ teaspoon kosher salt

1 teaspoon fresh lemon juice

½ teaspoon fresh ground black pepper

Method:

Wash green onions and slice green and white parts separately. Mince ginger and garlic.

Place skillet over medium flame and heat coconut oil until hot. Add white parts of green onions, ginger and garlic together. Sauté until brown for 1 minute. Add chopped coriander and cook one more minute.

Add shrimps and toss to coat. Season with salt and continue tossing for 3-4 minutes.

Stir in sliced green pieces of green onions and cook for 15 seconds. Season with lemon juice and pepper. Serve hot.

Nutritional Info:

Carbohydrates: 8g

Fats: 14.1g

Protein: 32.1g

Sugar:1.7g

iii) **Fish Steaks:**

Serving (s): 6

Ingredients:

6 thick salmon steaks

2 onions

1 green bell pepper

5 tomatoes

7 tablespoons extra virgin coconut oil

½ cup Coconut Cream Concentrate

3 tablespoons chopped parsley

3 tablespoons chopped fresh cilantro

¾ teaspoon hot red pepper

1 tablespoon salt

2 tablespoons lemon juice

Method:

Wash fish and pat dry. Place steaks into a shallow dish and season with salt and lemon juice. Allow steaks to marinade for 15 minutes.

Meanwhile, skinned onion and slice thinly. Slice bell pepper and tomatoes. Place skillet over medium flame and heat 3 tablespoons coconut oil until hot. Add onion and sauté until brown. Now add green pepper and fry for 3 more minutes. Add tomatoes in the skillet and cook for 2 minutes.

Now place fish steaks in the skillet and top it with remaining coconut oil. Cover the pan and cook the fish until cooked through. Uncover, and then add cilantro, parsley, and red pepper. Switch flame to high flame and cook until little liquid remains.

Add coconut cream and bring the dish to boil. Switch off the flame and transfer the dish in the serving bowl. Top with cilantro and serve hot.

Nutritional Info:

Carbohydrates: 3g

Fats: 12g

Protein: 19g

Sugar: 0g

b) Baking

The following baking recipes will surely melt in your mouth.

i) Coconut Oil Biscuits:

Serving (s): 6-8

Ingredients:

½ cup solid refined coconut oil

¾ cup canned light coconut milk

2 cups all-purpose flour

1 tablespoon baking powder

2 ½ teaspoons sugar

Method:

Preheat oven to 200 degrees C and line the baking sheet with aluminum foil or parchment paper. Microwave solid coconut oil for 4-5 seconds until soften, not runny.

In a large mixing bowl, mix flour, baking powder, salt and sugar together. Add coconut oil and mix using pastry blender until the mixture resembles crumbs.

Pour in coconut milk and stir until mixture forms into a light dough.

Clean the working space and floured liberally.

Transfer the biscuit mix to the working place and flatten using a rolling pin into a rectangle dough about half inch.

Cut into biscuits using a cookie cutter and place them on the lined baking sheet with an inch distance between them.

Brush the biscuits with coconut milk and sprinkle sugar.

Transfer baking sheet into the preheated oven and bake until golden for 18-20 minutes.

Place them on the cooling rack for 10 minutes before serving.

Nutritional Info:

Carbohydrates: 17g

Fats: 10g

Protein: 2g

Sugar: 0.5g

ii)   **Coconut Oil Chocolate Chip Cookies:**

Serving (s): 6-8

Ingredients:

½ cup coconut oil

½ cup granulated sugar

½ cup light brown sugar, packed

1 egg

1 ½ teaspoons vanilla extract

1 cup all-purpose flour

¾ cup all-purpose flour

1 teaspoon baking soda

1 cup white chocolate chips

1 cup nuts (of your choice), roughly chopped

Method:

Microwave solid coconut oil for 4-5 seconds until soften, not runny.

In a bowl, crack egg, add sugar, vanilla together and beat with pastry blender on a medium high speed for 5 minutes until fluffy and combined.

Scrap down the sides using plastic spatula and add flour, baking soda and salt.

Mix with pastry blender for a minute until combined well.

Now fold in white chocolates and nuts.

Use cookie scoop to form heap mounds of cookie mix on a large plate, keep an inch distance between them.

Now cover the plate with a cling film or plastic wrap and place in the fridge for three hours.

Meanwhile, preheat oven to 350 degree F and line baking tray with parchment and spray lightly with coconut oil.

Take the cookie dough from the fridge and place on the baking sheet with a 2 inch distance between them.

Place the baking sheet in the medium rack of the preheated oven and bake for 11-13 minutes until set and glossy.

Place them on the cooling rack for 10 minutes before serving.

Nutritional Info:

Carbohydrates: 17.9g

Fats: 9.4g

Protein: 1.3g

Sugar: 9.6g

iii) **Baked Chicken Tenders:**

Serving (s): 6

Ingredients:

1 boneless and skinless chicken breast

½ cup shredded coconut

¼ cup coconut oil

½ teaspoon salt

¼ teaspoon ground black pepper

¾ cup flour

2 eggs

2 teaspoons soy sauce

1 ¼ cups bread crumbs

Method:

Preheat oven to 400 degrees F.

Wash chicken breast and pat dry. Cut into bite size pieces on a cutting board.

Transfer chicken pieces into a shallow dish and season with salt and pepper and allow to marinate for 15-20 minutes.

Meanwhile, in a shallow dish, place flour. In a mixing bowl, crack eggs and add soy sauce, mix well.

In another shallow dish, place coconut and bread crumbs and mix.

Coat each chicken piece in flour and then dip into egg mix and transfer into the breadcrumbs-coconut mixture.

Dredge the chicken piece in the mixture.

Shake off the excess and place in a plate. Coat the remaining chicken pieces in the same way.

Heat a skillet over medium high flame and add coconut oil.

Fry chicken pieces in a single layer until golden brown for 3-4 minutes. Transfer fried chicken to the baking sheet and place into the preheated oven.

Bake for 10 minutes until cooked through. Serve hot with chilli sauce.

Nutritional Info:

Carbohydrates: 1.9g

Fats: 0g

Protein: 24g

Sugar: 0g

c) **Other Recipes**
i) **Coffee/Tea**

What's the first thing that comes into your mind when you wake up? Coffee or tea. No one can start a day without a warming savory beverage. This is a very simple yet an important way to start a day so why don't you add coconut oil in your coffee to make it more flavorful and refreshing. Or have it mid-day to energize you.

Refreshing Herbal Coffee/Tea:

Serving (s): 1

Ingredients:

1 cup of herbal coffee or green tea

1 or 2 tablespoons coconut oil

½ teaspoon vanilla

Method:

In a cup, add boiling water to either coffee or tea.

Add 1 or 2 tablespoons of coconut oil.

Stir well, Enjoy it!

Nutritional Info:

Carbohydrates: 2g

Fats: 0g

Protein: 0g

Sugar: 1g

ii)Banana Ice Cream:

Serving (s): 3-4

Ingredients:

20 pitted dates

2 tablespoons raw honey

2 tablespoons extra virgin coconut oil

1 teaspoon vanilla extract

1/8 teaspoon ground cinnamon

4 cups sliced very ripe bananas

1/2 cup raw peanuts

2 tablespoons cacao nibs

Method:

First, roughly chop dates and raw peanuts.

Soak the chopped dates in some warm water for 10 minutes. Drain and reserve the liquid.

Meanwhile, in a food processor, blend the dates, 4 tablespoons of the liquid, honey, coconut oil, vanilla extract, cinnamon together until smooth. Now transfer this mixture into a freezer friendly container, add peanuts and cacao nibs.

Stir until combined, cover and place in the freezer for 5-6 hours until it is solid. Serve and enjoy.

Nutritional Info:

Carbohydrates: 27g

Fats: 0g, Protein: 3g and sugar 1.2g

iii)   Cacao Chip Coconut Sandwich Spread:

Serving (s): 2-3

5 tablespoons virgin coconut oil

1 teaspoon raw cacao nibs

½ banana

2 teaspoons cacao powder

dash of cinnamon

2 teaspoons maple syrup

pinch of salt

Method:

In a food processor, add coconut oil, cacao nibs, cacao powder, banana, cinnamon, maple syrup and salt. Blend until creamy.

Spoon the spread in the freezer friendly container and place in the freezer for 15 minutes.

Nutritional Info:

Carbohydrates: 7g

Fats: 13g

Protein: 3g

Sugar: 8g

FINAL THOUGHTS ON COCONUT OIL

There is no doubt that coconut oil is fast becoming more popular than it was so many years back. With the new and more researches, studies, verifications and experiments on coconut oil people are becoming more aware of the immense contributions of the oil to their health and general wellbeing. It is now obvious that the healthy fatty acids in coconut oil and its enormous unique properties make it stand out amongst vegetable and other edible oils as well as an effective super food and remedy in the medical treatments. All these have made people to refer to Coconut oil as the "**MIRACLE OIL",** while in the Philippines; it is referred to as **"THE DRUGSTORE IN A BOTTLE"**